THE COMPLETE EASY LOW-FODMAP DIET RECIPES AND MEAL PLAN: 2024 Edition

"Revitalizing Your Digestive Health with Tasty and Digestion-Friendly Meals"

Liam Bryce

Table of Contents:

INTRODUCTION

There once lived a lively woman named Bryce in the thriving town of Evergreen. Food had always been Bryce's passion, and her desire to help people have better, more satisfying lives was even more intense than her love of cooking. It never occurred to her that her path would result in the publication of the groundbreaking cookbook "Complete Easy Low-FODMAP Diet Recipes and Meal Plan: 2024 Edition."

Bryce had endured years of suffering from intestinal problems, never knowing what meals would set off her misery. Exasperated by the dearth of useful materials at her disposal, she set out to find a way that would help her and many others who were going through similar struggles.

After years of unrelenting investigation and testing, Bryce came onto the Low-FODMAP diet, a dietary strategy intended to reduce symptoms associated with irritable bowel syndrome (IBS) and other gastrointestinal disorders. She was driven to share her research with the world after seeing the wonderful effects of this new eating style on her own life.

Bryce, meanwhile, wanted to do more than just provide a list of things that were off-limits and unclear restrictions. She was aware that individuals required an all-inclusive guide to easily manage the complexity of the low-FODMAP diet. So she started working on a cookbook that would include delicious dishes and a well-thought-out food plan.

Her vision's realization was not without some difficulties. In her little kitchen, Bryce experimented for hours on end with different ingredients and combinations to produce delicious dishes that were also easy on the stomach. She worked with elite chefs and nutritionists to make sure every recipe was the best it could be in terms of both flavor and nutrition.

Bryce knew, though, that a cookbook by itself would not suffice. She desired for her idea to have a genuine impact on individuals and provide them with a sense of belonging and support. Consequently, she decided to intertwine narratives throughout the book, offering tales and insights from both her personal experience and those of others who had discovered comfort in the Low-FODMAP diet.

This book, "Complete Easy Low-FODMAP Diet Recipes and Meal Plan: 2024 Edition," will take readers to cozy, humorous kitchens. Stories of tenacity, victory, and the happiness of living again without experiencing stomach pain would be told to them. Each reader felt encouraged and understood thanks to Bryce's narration.

The cookbook took off, becoming well-known not just in Evergreen, Colorado, but also all around the world. Numerous people were inspired to adopt the Low-FODMAP diet and experience a revitalized feeling of energy and well-being by Bryce's commitment, compassion, and love of food, which had started a movement.

When starting the Low-FODMAP diet, folks no longer felt overwhelmed since they had her cookbook. By demonstrating that a restricted diet could still be tasty and fulfilling, Bryce's dishes turned their mealtimes into happy and meaningful occasions Anyone may easily follow along and profit from the meal plan as it offers structure and direction.

As the author of the "Complete Easy Low-FODMAP Diet Recipes and Meal Plan: 2024 Edition," Bryce leaves behind a lasting legacy that encourages the next generations to choose better lifestyles. Her experience serves as a reminder that we may positively impact lives and change how we handle dietary limitations by being compassionate and hardworking.

The Low-FODMAP diet is a dietary approach designed to manage symptoms of certain gastrointestinal disorders, such as irritable bowel syndrome (IBS). FODMAPs are a group of fermentable carbohydrates that can trigger digestive symptoms in some individuals. The acronym stands for Fermentable Oligosaccharides, Disaccharides, Monosaccharides, and Polyols. By following a Low-FODMAP diet, individuals can identify and avoid these specific types of carbohydrates, potentially reducing their symptoms and improving their quality of life.

Concept of the Low-FODMAP diet:

The concept behind the Low-FODMAP diet is to limit the intake of specific carbohydrates that are poorly absorbed by the small intestine. When these carbohydrates reach the large intestine, gut bacteria ferment them, leading to the production of gas, which can cause symptoms like bloating, abdominal pain, flatulence, diarrhea, and constipation.

The Low-FODMAP diet involves three key phases: the elimination phase, the reintroduction phase, and the personalization phase.

Elimination phase: During this phase, individuals strictly avoid high-FODMAP foods for a period of 2-6 weeks. This aims to reduce symptoms and provide symptom relief.

Reintroduction phase: In this phase, high-FODMAP foods are gradually reintroduced one at a time, in specific quantities and intervals, while monitoring symptoms. This step helps identify individual sensitivities to specific FODMAP groups.

Personalization phase: Using the information gathered during the reintroduction phase, individuals can create a personalized, long-term diet plan. This phase involves maintaining a balance by avoiding high-FODMAP foods that trigger symptoms while incorporating a variety of low-FODMAP foods into everyday meals.

Benefits of the Low-FODMAP diet:

The Low-FODMAP diet has shown promising results in managing symptoms associated with digestive disorders, particularly IBS. Benefits of this dietary approach may include:

Symptom relief: By avoiding high-FODMAP foods, individuals often experience reductions in bloating, abdominal pain, diarrhea, and constipation. This can lead to an overall improvement in quality of life.

Individual customization: The reintroduction phase allows individuals to understand their specific triggers, helping them create a personalized diet plan that suits their needs and preferences.

Increased dietary diversity: Despite the restrictions, the Low-FODMAP diet can still include a wide variety of low-FODMAP foods, ensuring nutritional adequacy and preventing monotony in meals.

Identification of trigger foods: By reintroducing high-FODMAP foods systematically, individuals can identify specific FODMAP groups that cause symptoms, enabling them to make informed choices about their diet in the long term.

It's important to note that the Low-FODMAP diet is best undertaken with the guidance of a registered dietitian or healthcare professional, as it requires careful monitoring and supervision to ensure proper nutritional balance and individualized management.

Importance of maintaining a balanced diet for digestive health

Maintaining a balanced diet is crucial for promoting and maintaining good digestive health. The digestive system is responsible for breaking down food, absorbing nutrients, and eliminating waste. When we consume a balanced diet, it provides the necessary nutrients and fiber to keep our digestive system functioning optimally. Here are some key reasons why a balanced diet is important for digestive health:

Nutrient absorption: A balanced diet ensures that the body receives an adequate amount of essential nutrients such as carbohydrates, proteins, fats, vitamins, and minerals. These nutrients are essential for the proper digestion and absorption of food. For example, fiber aids in digestion by adding bulk to the stool and preventing constipation. A diet lacking in these nutrients may lead to digestive issues like malabsorption or nutrient deficiencies.

Gut microbiota health: The gut microbiota refers to the trillions of bacteria and other microorganisms that reside in our digestive system. These beneficial bacteria help with digestion, produce certain vitamins, strengthen the immune system, and maintain a healthy gut environment. A balanced diet with plenty of fruits, vegetables, whole grains, and fermented foods nourishes the gut microbiota, promoting a diverse and balanced composition. This is important for a healthy digestive system and overall well-being.

Bowel regularity: Adequate fiber intake is crucial for maintaining regular bowel movements. Fiber adds bulk to the stool, promotes efficient movement through the digestive tract, and prevents constipation. A balanced diet rich in fruits, vegetables, whole grains, and legumes provides ample fiber, helping to regulate bowel movements and prevent digestive issues like constipation and hemorrhoids.

Digestive disorder prevention: A balanced diet can help prevent various digestive disorders. For instance, excessive intake of high-fat, processed foods can increase the risk of developing conditions like gallstones, gastroesophageal reflux disease (GERD), and inflammatory bowel diseases (IBD). On the other hand, a diet rich in fiber and low in processed foods can lower the risk of developing conditions like diverticulosis, hemorrhoids, and gastrointestinal cancers.

Weight management: Achieving and maintaining a healthy weight is essential for digestive health. An imbalanced diet high in unhealthy fats, sugars, and processed foods can lead to weight gain, obesity, and an increased risk of developing conditions such as fatty liver disease, heartburn, and acid reflux. On the other hand, a balanced diet that includes lean proteins, whole grains, fruits, vegetables, and healthy fats promotes weight management, reducing the risk of digestive disorders.

Overview of the 2024 edition updates and improvements

The 2024 edition of the Complete Easy Low-FODMAP Diet Recipes and Meal Plan brings significant updates and improvements designed to support individuals adhering to a low-FODMAP diet. This edition focuses on providing delicious and diverse recipes while ensuring easy preparation and accessibility.

Some key updates and improvements include:

Updated food lists: The edition features an updated list of low-FODMAP foods, making it easier for individuals to select safe ingredients for their meals. It includes a wide range of fruits, vegetables, proteins, grains, and snacks that can be incorporated into a low-FODMAP diet.

Increased variety: The meal plan offers a wider variety of recipes to prevent monotony and meet the nutritional needs of individuals. It includes different cuisines, flavors, and cooking techniques, ensuring a diverse and enjoyable eating experience.

Enhanced nutritional information: Each recipe is accompanied by detailed nutritional information, including macronutrients and portion sizes, helping individuals keep track of their intake and make informed decisions about their diet.

Quick and easy meal options: The 2024 edition recognizes the need for convenience in everyday cooking. It features a section dedicated to quick and easy low-FODMAP meals, providing options for busy individuals who don't have much time to cook.

Healthful snacks and treats: The book now includes a selection of low-FODMAP snacks and treats to satisfy cravings without compromising the diet. These options ensure individuals can still enjoy a variety of delicious goodies while adhering to the low-FODMAP guidelines.

Dietary substitution suggestions: The edition provides helpful substitution suggestions for common ingredients to accommodate dietary restrictions or preferences, making it easier to adapt recipes to individual needs.

Comprehensive meal plans: The updated edition includes comprehensive meal plans for different dietary preferences, such as vegetarian or gluten-free options. These plans help individuals structure their meals effectively and ensure a balanced approach to their low-FODMAP diet.

Tips for dining out: Recognizing that eating out can be a challenge, the book offers practical tips for navigating restaurants and social gatherings while following a low-FODMAP diet. It provides guidance on reading menus, making suitable choices, and communicating dietary needs to servers.

The 2024 edition of the Complete Easy Low-FODMAP Diet Recipes and Meal Plan strives to be an invaluable resource for anyone following a low-FODMAP diet. With its updated recipes, meal plans, and guidance, individuals can confidently manage their diet while enjoying delicious and satisfying meals.

UNDERSTANDING THE LOW-FODMAP DIET

FODMAPs and their relationship to digestive issues

FODMAPs (Fermentable Oligosaccharides, Disaccharides, Monosaccharides, and Polyols) are a group of carbohydrates found in certain foods. These carbohydrates can be poorly absorbed in the small intestine, leading to their fermentation by bacteria in the large intestine. This fermentation process can cause digestive issues in some individuals, especially those who are sensitive or intolerant to FODMAPs.

Component of FODMAPs:

Fermentable: FODMAPs are easily fermented by the gut bacteria in the large intestine. During fermentation, gases such as hydrogen, methane, and carbon dioxide are produced. The build-up of these gases can contribute to symptoms like bloating, flatulence, and abdominal discomfort.

Oligosaccharides: This category includes fructans and galacto-oligosaccharides (GOS). Fructans are found in foods like wheat, rye, barley, onions, garlic, and some fruits and vegetables. GOS are present in legumes, such as beans and lentils. Oligosaccharides are not well absorbed in the small intestine, and when fermented in the large intestine, they can cause symptoms in sensitive individuals.

Disaccharides: Lactose, the primary disaccharide, is found in dairy products. Some individuals have a deficiency of lactase, the enzyme responsible for breaking down lactose. This leads to lactose intolerance, as undigested lactose can cause gastrointestinal symptoms when it reaches the large intestine.

Monosaccharides: Fructose, a monosaccharide, is found in high amounts in honey, fruits like apples and pears, and some sweeteners like high fructose corn syrup. When consumed in excess of glucose, fructose can be poorly absorbed in the small intestine and can cause symptoms in those who are fructose intolerant.

Polyols: These are sugar alcohols like sorbitol, mannitol, xylitol, and maltitol, often used as sweeteners in sugar-free gums, candies, and some fruits. Polyols have osmotic properties, meaning they draw water into the intestine, leading to diarrhea and other digestive discomforts in some individuals.

The relationship between FODMAPs and digestive issues is complex. For individuals with irritable bowel syndrome (IBS), some studies have shown that a low FODMAP diet can reduce symptoms like bloating, gas, abdominal pain, and altered bowel habits. However, it's important to note that FODMAPs are not the cause of IBS but can worsen symptoms in susceptible individuals.

If you suspect you have issues with FODMAPs, it's best to consult with a healthcare professional, preferably a registered dietitian with expertise in the low FODMAP diet. They can help you identify trigger foods, guide you through the elimination phase, and provide strategies for reintroducing FODMAPs back into your diet.

Low-FODMAP diet and how it can help alleviate symptoms

The Low-FODMAP diet is an evidence-based approach that targets the management of symptoms related to irritable bowel syndrome (IBS) and other digestive disorders. FODMAPs (Fermentable Oligosaccharides, Disaccharides, Monosaccharides, and Polyols) are a group of carbohydrates that are poorly absorbed by the small intestine, leading to increased water content and gas production in the colon, resulting in symptoms like bloating, abdominal pain, and changes in bowel movements. The principles of the Low-FODMAP diet are as follows:

Elimination Phase: The first phase involves the complete removal of high-FODMAP foods from the diet for a specific period, typically 2-6 weeks. This phase allows for symptom relief and helps identify if FODMAPs are the triggering factor for the symptoms. High-FODMAP foods include wheat, garlic, onions, certain fruits (such as apples, cherries, and pears), lactose-containing dairy products, legumes, and sweeteners like honey and high-fructose corn syrup.

Reintroduction Phase: In this phase, individual FODMAP groups are gradually reintroduced systematically, one at a time, while closely monitoring symptoms. This step identifies which specific types of FODMAPs trigger symptoms and to what extent. It helps build a personalized understanding of which

FODMAPs an individual can tolerate and in what quantities.

Personalization Phase: Once the high-FODMAP food triggers are identified, this phase focuses on personalizing the diet based on the individual's tolerance levels. Not all high-FODMAP foods trigger symptoms in everyone, and some may tolerate certain FODMAPs in small amounts. This phase aims to create a balanced diet that minimizes symptom triggers while maintaining nutritional adequacy.

Benefits of the Low-FODMAP diet:

- Reduced symptoms: Studies have shown that the Low-FODMAP diet can significantly reduce symptoms like bloating, abdominal pain, and altered bowel movements in individuals with IBS and other digestive disorders.

- Increased control: Following a Low-FODMAP diet empowers individuals by allowing them to identify their specific triggers and make informed dietary choices to manage their symptoms effectively.

- Improved quality of life: By alleviating symptoms, the Low-FODMAP diet can improve overall quality of life, reducing the impact of digestive symptoms on daily activities and well-being.

- Personalized approach: The reintroduction and personalization phases of the diet help individuals personalize their diet to their specific needs, ensuring they are not overly restricted but find a balance that works for them.

It's important to note that the Low-FODMAP diet should be undertaken under the guidance of a healthcare professional, such as a registered dietitian, to ensure the diet is followed correctly and nutritional needs are met.

Types of FODMAPs and their sources

FODMAPs, which stands for Fermentable Oligosaccharides, Disaccharides, Monosaccharides, and Polyols, are a group of short-chain carbohydrates that can cause digestive discomfort in some individuals. They are classified into several types, each with its own sources.

Types of FODMAPs and examples of their sources:

Oligosaccharides:

- Fructans: Found in wheat, rye, barley, onions, garlic, artichokes, asparagus, leeks, and some fruits like apples and pears.
- Fructo-oligosaccharides (FOS): Added to many processed foods as a prebiotic and also found naturally in some vegetables and legumes.

Disaccharides:

- Lactose: Found in dairy products such as milk, yogurt, and soft cheeses.

Monosaccharides:

- Fructose: Found in high amounts in honey, apples, pears, mangoes, and certain sweeteners like high-fructose corn syrup.
- High-fructose fruits: Some fruits like watermelon, cherries, and blackberries contain higher levels of fructose.

Polyols:

- Sorbitol: Found naturally in some fruits (e.g., apples, pears) and added as a sweetener in certain foods.
- Mannitol: Present in mushrooms, cauliflower, and sweeteners like xylitol.
- Xylitol: Commonly used as a sugar substitute in chewing gums, candies, and some processed foods.
- Maltitol, isomalt, and other sugar alcohols: Found in some sugar-free products.

It's important to note that FODMAP content can vary within food categories, different ripeness levels, and sources. Some individuals may have sensitivities to specific FODMAP types, while others may react to multiple types. If experiencing digestive issues, it is advisable to consult with a healthcare professional or a registered dietitian who can provide personalized guidance on a low FODMAP diet.

CREATING YOUR MEAL PLAN

High-FODMAP foods and ingredients from your diet

Eliminating high-FODMAP foods and ingredients from your diet can be a helpful strategy if you're experiencing symptoms of irritable bowel syndrome (IBS) or other digestive issues related to FODMAP sensitivity. FODMAPs are a group of fermentable carbohydrates that can trigger digestive symptoms in certain individuals. It's important to note that following a low-FODMAP diet should be done under the guidance of a registered dietitian or healthcare professional. Some general steps you can take to eliminate high-FODMAP foods from your diet:

Educate yourself: Learn about the different types of FODMAPs and which foods are high in each category. Common high-FODMAP foods include certain fruits, vegetables, grains, dairy products, sweeteners, and certain legumes.

Keep a food diary: Before starting the elimination phase, it can be helpful to keep a food diary to track your symptoms and identify any patterns. This will give you a baseline to compare against once you start eliminating high-FODMAP foods.

Start with elimination: Begin by removing all high-FODMAP foods and ingredients from your diet for a period of 2-6 weeks. This phase is different for everyone, and the duration may vary based on your symptoms and professional guidance.

Monitor your symptoms: During the elimination phase, pay close attention to how your body responds. Keep track of symptoms, improvements, and any changes in your well-being.

Gradual reintroduction: After the elimination phase, you will reintroduce FODMAP foods back into your diet, one type at a time, in controlled amounts. This step helps determine your individual tolerance to each FODMAP group. A dietitian can guide you through this process while monitoring your symptoms.

Personalize your diet: Once you identify specific trigger foods, work with a dietitian to develop a personalized low-FODMAP diet plan. This plan should eliminate or limit high-FODMAP foods while still providing a balanced and nutritious diet.

Seek professional guidance: It's important to consult a registered dietitian or healthcare professional who specializes in the low-FODMAP diet. They can help you navigate the elimination and reintroduction phases, ensure you maintain adequate nutrition, and adjust the plan to suit your individual needs.

The low-FODMAP diet is not meant to be followed long-term. The goal is to identify your trigger foods and establish a diet that avoids high-FODMAP foods while still maintaining a healthy and well-rounded eating plan. This ensures you have a sustainable and enjoyable way of eating without compromising your digestive health.

Keeping Food diary to track symptoms and dietary changes

Keeping a food diary can be a valuable tool for tracking symptoms and dietary changes, especially for individuals who suffer from certain health conditions or are seeking specific health goals. It involves recording everything you eat and drink, as well as any symptoms or changes you experience as a result. Reasons why keeping a food diary is important:

Identifying food intolerance or allergies: Some individuals may be sensitive or allergic to certain foods but aren't aware of it. By consistently recording your diet and noting any symptoms that occur, you can start to notice patterns and potential trigger foods. This information can be very helpful in identifying food intolerances or allergies, which in turn can help you adjust your diet accordingly and eliminate problematic foods.

Managing chronic conditions: People with chronic conditions such as irritable bowel syndrome (IBS), Crohn's disease, or diabetes often find it beneficial to keep a food diary. These conditions can be affected by the foods you consume, and tracking your diet can help you identify specific triggers or problematic food groups. By keeping a record of your symptoms alongside your dietary choices, you can make informed decisions about which foods to avoid or include in your meals to better manage your condition.

Assessing the impact of dietary changes: If you're making changes to your diet, such as trying out a new meal plan, eliminating certain foods, or introducing more nutritious options, a food diary can help you evaluate the effects of these changes. By documenting what you eat and how you feel, you can determine if the dietary modifications are having the desired impact on your health, energy levels, weight, or other relevant factors.

Enhancing accountability and motivation: A food diary can act as a daily reminder of your health goals and provide accountability. It forces you to think more consciously about your food choices, making you less likely to mindlessly snack on unhealthy options. In addition, the act of writing down your meals and symptoms can help motivate you to stick to your dietary plan and make healthier choices in the long run.

Facilitating discussions with healthcare professionals: If you're seeing a healthcare professional, sharing your food diary with them can provide valuable information for diagnosis and treatment. A detailed record of your eating patterns and symptoms can assist your healthcare provider in better understanding your condition and making appropriate recommendations. It can also help you and your healthcare team spot potential nutrient deficiencies or imbalances that may need attention.

Keeping a food diary offers several advantages when it comes to tracking symptoms and dietary changes. It can help identify food intolerances, manage chronic conditions, assess the impact of dietary modifications, enhance accountability, and facilitate discussions with healthcare professionals. By consistently recording your food intake and symptoms, you can gain valuable insights into your body's response to different foods and make informed choices to support your health and well-being.

Meal planning and grocery shopping on the Low-FODMAP diet

Meal planning and grocery shopping on the Low-FODMAP diet:

Understand the Low-FODMAP diet: Familiarize yourself with the foods that are high and low in FODMAPs. FODMAPs are certain types of carbohydrates that can trigger digestive symptoms in some individuals.

Plan your meals: Start by creating a meal plan for the week. This will help you stay organized and ensure that you have suitable options available. Consider including a variety of low-FODMAP fruits, vegetables, grains, proteins, and fats.

Find low-FODMAP recipes: Look for recipes that are specifically designed for the Low-FODMAP diet. Use cookbooks, websites, or smart phone apps to discover new ideas and meal inspiration.

Make a grocery list: Once you have your meal plan, make a detailed grocery list. This will help you stay focused and avoid purchasing items that are high in FODMAPs. Categorize your list according to different food groups to make shopping easier.

Read food labels: When shopping, carefully read the food labels to identify high-FODMAP ingredients. Common high-FODMAP ingredients include wheat, honey, garlic, onions, and high-fructose corn syrup.

Opt for products labeled as "low-FODMAP" or check for ingredients that are safe for consumption.

Stock up on low-FODMAP staples: Keep your pantry stocked with low-FODMAP staples such as gluten-free grains (rice, quinoa), canned tomatoes, herbs, spices, olive oil, lactose-free dairy products, and suitable snacks.

Shop the perimeter: The outer aisles of the grocery store typically contain fresh produce, meats, and dairy products, which are generally low in FODMAPs. Focus on these sections of the store when shopping.

Experiment with new foods: Use this opportunity to try new low-FODMAP ingredients you might not have consumed before, such as quinoa, tofu, or specific gluten-free grains.

Consider batch cooking: If you have limited time during the week, spend a few hours on the weekend batch cooking meals and prepping ingredients. This can save time and make it easier to stick to your low-FODMAP diet.

Stay organized: Keep your pantry, fridge, and freezer organized to quickly locate low-FODMAP ingredients and avoid any cross-contamination with high-FODMAP foods.

BREAKFAST RECIPES

Variety of low-FODMAP breakfast options, including both savory and sweet dishes

Variety of low-FODMAP breakfast options that include both savory and sweet dishes:

Savory Omelette:

- Spinach and feta cheese omelette with a side of roasted cherry tomatoes.
- Mushroom and cheddar cheese omelette with a side of sautéed zucchini.

Sweet Potato Toast:

- Toasted slices of sweet potato topped with almond butter and sliced banana.
- Sweet potato toast topped with mashed avocado and a sprinkle of chili flakes.

Quinoa Breakfast Bowl:

- Cooked quinoa topped with mixed berries, a dollop of lactose-free yogurt, and a drizzle of maple syrup.
- Quinoa with roasted butternut squash, spinach, and a sprinkle of feta cheese.

Banana Pancakes:

- Mix mashed banana with gluten-free oats, eggs, and a pinch of cinnamon. Cook like regular pancakes and serve with a drizzle of maple syrup.
- Add blueberries or strawberries to the pancake batter for added flavor.

Greek Yogurt Parfait:

- Layer lactose-free Greek yogurt, low-FODMAP granola, and sliced strawberries in a glass.

Repeat the layers and top with a spoonful of nut butter.

- Use lactose-free Greek yogurt, chopped kiwi, and toasted coconut flakes for a tropical twist.

Breakfast Burrito/Bowl:

- Scramble eggs with sautéed bell peppers, spinach, and lactose-free cheese. Wrap in a gluten-free tortilla or serve over a bed of rice.
- Create a bowl using scrambled eggs, cooked quinoa, sautéed zucchini, and a spoonful of salsa.

Smoothie:

- Blueberry Banana Smoothie: Blend frozen blueberries, ripe banana, lactose-free milk, and a spoonful of peanut butter.
- Tropical Green Smoothie: Blend spinach, pineapple, kiwi, coconut milk, and a handful of ice.

Quiche:

- Make a gluten-free quiche using a crust made from almond flour or a mixture of gluten-free flours. Fill it with low-FODMAP veggies like spinach, bell peppers, and diced tomatoes. Add lactose-free cheese and eggs as the base. Bake until set and golden.

Chia Seed Pudding:

- Mix chia seeds with lactose-free milk, a dash of vanilla extract, and a sweetener like maple syrup or stevia. Let it sit in the refrigerator overnight to thicken. Serve topped with low-FODMAP fruits like strawberries, kiwi, or raspberries.

Breakfast Wrap:

- Use a gluten-free wrap or lettuce leaves as a base. Fill it with scrambled eggs, cooked bacon (without garlic or onion), sliced avocado, and tomato. Add a dollop of lactose-free sour cream or mayo if desired.

Buckwheat Pancakes:

- Make pancakes using buckwheat flour (a low-FODMAP alternative). Mix it with lactose-free milk, eggs, and a bit of baking powder. Cook on a non-stick pan and enjoy with a drizzle of maple syrup or low-FODMAP fruit compote.

Frittata:

- Whisk eggs with lactose-free milk and seasonings. Sauté low-FODMAP veggies like zucchini, bell peppers, and spinach. Pour the egg mixture over the vegetables in a pan and cook until set. Serve as individual slices or refrigerate for later use.

Rice Cakes with Toppings:

- Use rice cakes as a gluten-free base. Top them with options like lactose-free cream cheese, smoked salmon, cucumber slices, and dill. You can also try mashed avocado, sliced hard-boiled eggs, and cherry tomatoes.

Overnight Oats:

- Use gluten-free oats and mix with lactose-free milk, chia seeds, and your choice of low-FODMAP toppings like sliced banana, almonds, and a drizzle of maple syrup. Let it sit overnight in the refrigerator for a quick and easy breakfast.

Shakshuka:

- Make a low-FODMAP shakshuka using a tomato sauce base, mixed with bell peppers and spices like cumin, paprika, and cayenne pepper. Poach eggs directly in the sauce and serve with gluten-free bread or a side of rice.

These breakfast options provide a range of flavors and ingredients to suit your preferences. Remember to always double-check the ingredient labels and serving sizes to ensure they align with your low-FODMAP diet.

Easy-to-follow recipes for delicious meals

Easy-to-follow recipes for a FODMAP-friendly omelet, overnight chia pudding, and grain-free pancakes:

FODMAP-Friendly Omelet:

Ingredients:

- 2 large eggs
- 1/4 cup lactose-free milk
- 1/4 cup diced bell peppers (red, yellow, or orange)
- 1/4 cup diced zucchini
- 1 tablespoon chopped chives
- Salt and pepper to taste

- Olive oil or lactose-free butter for cooking

Instructions:

1. In a bowl, whisk the eggs and milk together until well combined. Season with salt and pepper.

2. Heat a small non-stick skillet over medium heat and add a drizzle of olive oil or lactose-free butter.

3. Add the diced bell peppers and zucchini to the skillet and sauté for about 2 minutes until slightly softened.

4. Pour the egg mixture into the skillet over the vegetables. Sprinkle chopped chives on top.

5. Cook the omelet for about 2-3 minutes until the bottom is set. Flip the omelet using a spatula and cook for an additional 1-2 minutes.

6. Slide the omelet onto a plate, fold it in half, and serve hot.

Overnight Chia Pudding:

Ingredients:

- 2 tablespoons chia seeds
- 1/2 cup lactose-free milk or non-dairy alternative (e.g., almond milk)
- 1 tablespoon maple syrup (optional)
- 1/4 teaspoon vanilla extract
- Fresh berries for topping

Instructions:

1. In a jar or bowl, combine chia seeds, lactose-free milk, maple syrup (if desired), and vanilla extract. Stir well to combine.

2. Cover the jar or bowl and refrigerate overnight or for at least 4 hours until the chia seeds have absorbed the liquid and the mixture thickens.

3. Give the chia pudding a good stir to break up any clumps. If it's too thick, you can add a little more milk.

4. Serve the chia pudding in bowls or glasses and top with fresh berries. Enjoy it cold.

Grain-Free Pancakes:

Ingredients:

- 1 ripe banana
- 2 large eggs
- 1/4 teaspoon vanilla extract
- 1/4 teaspoon ground cinnamon
- Cooking oil or butter for greasing the pan

Instructions:

1. In a bowl, mash the ripe banana until smooth.

2. Add the eggs, vanilla extract, and ground cinnamon to the bowl. Whisk everything together until well combined.

3. Heat a non-stick skillet or griddle over medium heat and grease it with cooking oil or butter.

4. Pour about 1/4 cup of the pancake batter onto the skillet for each pancake.

5. Cook for about 2-3 minutes until bubbles form on the surface. Flip the pancakes and cook for an additional 1-2 minutes until golden brown.

6. Serve the grain-free pancakes warm with your favorite toppings such as fresh fruits, maple syrup, or nut butter.

Quinoa Salad with Roasted Vegetables:

Ingredients:

- 1 cup quinoa
- 2 cups water or vegetable broth
- Assorted vegetables (such as bell peppers, zucchini, eggplant)
- Olive oil
- Salt and pepper to taste
- Fresh herbs (such as parsley or basil), chopped

- Lemon juice for dressing

Instructions:

1. Preheat the oven to 400°F (200°C).

2. Rinse the quinoa under cold water and drain.

3. In a medium saucepan, bring the water or vegetable broth to a boil. Add the quinoa and reduce heat to low. Cover and simmer for 15-20 minutes until the liquid is absorbed and the quinoa is tender. Remove from heat.

4. Meanwhile, chop the vegetables into bite-sized pieces and place them on a baking sheet. Drizzle with olive oil and season with salt and pepper.

5. Roast the vegetables in the preheated oven for about 20-25 minutes until they are tender and slightly caramelized.

6. In a large mixing bowl, combine the cooked quinoa and roasted vegetables. Add fresh herbs and toss gently.

7. Drizzle with lemon juice and adjust salt and pepper to taste. Serve warm or cold as a side dish or main course.

Stir-Fried Ginger Garlic Shrimp:

Ingredients:

- 1 pound shrimp, peeled and deveined
- 2 tablespoons soy sauce or tamari (gluten-free alternative)
- 1 tablespoon honey (optional)
- 1 tablespoon sesame oil
- 1 tablespoon fresh ginger, minced
- 2 cloves garlic, minced
- 2 tablespoons olive oil
- Assorted vegetables (such as bell peppers, snap peas, carrots)
- Green onions, sliced for garnish

Instructions:

1. In a bowl, combine soy sauce, honey, sesame oil, minced ginger, and minced garlic. Stir to combine and set aside.

2. Heat olive oil in a large skillet or wok over medium-high heat.

3. Add the shrimp to the hot skillet and cook for about 2 minutes per side until they turn pink and are slightly opaque. Remove shrimp from the skillet and set aside.

4. In the same skillet, add the vegetables and stir-fry for about 3-4 minutes until they are tender-crisp.

5. Return the shrimp to the skillet and pour the sauce over the shrimp and vegetables. Stir-fry for an additional 1-2 minutes until everything is coated and heated through.

6. Garnish with sliced green onions and serve hot over steamed rice or noodles.

Roasted Chicken with Root Vegetables:

Ingredients:

- 1 whole chicken, about 4-5 pounds

- Assorted root vegetables (such as carrots, parsnips, potatoes), peeled and sliced
- 2 tablespoons olive oil
- 1 tablespoon dried herbs (such as rosemary, thyme, or oregano)
- Salt and pepper to tast

Instructions:

1. Preheat the oven to 425°F (220°C).

2. Place the whole chicken in a roasting pan or baking dish.

3. In a small bowl, mix together olive oil, dried herbs, salt, and pepper. Brush this mixture over the chicken, making sure to coat all sides.

4. Arrange the sliced root vegetables around the chicken in the roasting pan.

5. Roast the chicken and vegetables in the preheated oven for about 1 hour and 20 minutes, or until the

chicken is golden brown and the internal temperature reaches 165°F (75°C).

6. Remove the chicken from the oven and let it rest for a few minutes before carving.

7. Serve the roasted chicken with the root vegetables as a delicious and hearty meal.

I hope these recipes inspire you to try new dishes and enjoy delicious meals!

LUNCH AND DINNER RECIPES

Low-FODMAP recipes suitable for lunches and dinners

Low-FODMAP recipes that you can enjoy for lunches and dinners:

Grilled Chicken Salad:

Ingredients:

- Grilled chicken breast (sliced)
- Mixed salad greens
- Cherry tomatoes (halved)
- Cucumber (sliced)
- Carrot (shredded)
- Red bell pepper (sliced)

- Olive oil and lemon juice dressing

Quinoa Stuffed Bell Peppers:

Ingredients:

- Bell peppers (halved and deseeded)
- Cooked quinoa
- Spinach (chopped)
- Zucchini (diced)
- Tomato (diced)
- Green onions (green parts only, sliced)
- Olive oil
- Salt and pepper to taste

Instructions:

1. Preheat the oven to 375°F (190°C).

2. In a skillet, heat olive oil and sauté the zucchini until tender.

3. In a mixing bowl, combine cooked quinoa, spinach, tomato, green onions, sautéed zucchini, salt, and pepper.

4. Stuff the bell peppers with the quinoa mixture.

5. Place the stuffed peppers on a baking sheet and bake for about 25-30 minutes or until the peppers are tender.

Baked Salmon with Roasted Vegetables:

Ingredients:

- Salmon fillets
- Carrots (cut into sticks)
- Zucchini (cut into rounds)
- Red bell pepper (sliced)
- Asparagus (trimmed)
- Olive oil
- Lemon juice
- Dried dill
- Salt and pepper to taste

Instructions:

1. Preheat the oven to 400°F (200°C).

2. Arrange the vegetables on a baking sheet, drizzle with olive oil, lemon juice, dried dill, salt, and pepper. Toss to coat.

3. Place the salmon fillets on top of the vegetables and season with salt, pepper, and dried dill.

4. Bake for about 12-15 minutes or until the salmon is cooked through and the vegetables are tender.

Low-FODMAP Chicken Stir-Fry:

Ingredients:

- Chicken breast (sliced)
- Bell peppers (sliced)
- Carrots (cut into strips)
- Green beans (trimmed)
- Bok choy (chopped)

- Gluten-free soy sauce (check FODMAP-friendly brands)
- Garlic-infused oil
- Sesame oil (optional)
- Salt and pepper to taste

Instructions:

1. In a wok or large pan, heat garlic-infused oil over medium-high heat.

2. Add the sliced chicken and cook until browned.

3. Add the bell peppers, carrots, green beans, and bok choy to the pan. Stir-fry until the vegetables are tender-crisp.

4. Season with gluten-free soy sauce, sesame oil (if desired), salt, and pepper.

5. Serve with steamed rice or quinoa.

Spinach and Feta Stuffed Chicken Breast:

Ingredients:

- Chicken breast (boneless and skinless)
- Spinach (chopped)
- Feta cheese (crumbled)
- Sun-dried tomatoes (chopped)
- Fresh basil leaves (chopped)
- Salt and pepper to taste

Instructions:

1. Preheat the oven to 375°F (190°C).

2. Cut a pocket lengthwise in each chicken breast.

3. In a bowl, mix the spinach, feta cheese, sun-dried tomatoes, and basil. Season with salt and pepper.

4. Stuff the chicken breasts with the spinach mixture.

5. Heat some olive oil in a skillet over medium heat. Sear the stuffed chicken breasts on both sides until golden brown.

6. Transfer the chicken to a baking dish and bake in the preheated oven for about 20-25 minutes or until cooked through.

Low-FODMAP Turkey Lettuce Wraps:

Ingredients:

- Ground turkey
- Butter lettuce leaves (washed and separated)
- Carrots (julienned)
- Red cabbage (shredded)
- Cucumber (sliced)
- Fresh cilantro leaves
- Lime wedges
- Low-FODMAP stir-fry sauce (check labels)

Instructions:

1. In a skillet, cook the ground turkey until browned and cooked through.

2. Stir in the low-FODMAP stir-fry sauce and cook for an additional 2-3 minutes.

3. To assemble, place a spoonful of the cooked turkey in a lettuce leaf, then top with carrots, cabbage, cucumber, cilantro leaves, and a squeeze of lime juice.

4. Roll up the lettuce leaf and secure with a toothpick if needed. Repeat for remaining lettuce leaves.

Lemon Herb Roasted Chicken:

Ingredients:

- Whole chicken (cleaned and patted dry)
- Lemon (sliced)
- Fresh rosemary sprigs
- Fresh thyme sprigs
- Olive oil
- Salt and pepper to taste

Instructions:

1. Preheat the oven to 425°F (220°C).

2. Place the chicken on a roasting pan or ovenproof dish.

3. Drizzle olive oil all over the chicken and season with salt and pepper.

4. Place lemon slices, rosemary sprigs, and thyme sprigs under the skin of the chicken and inside the cavity.

5. Roast the chicken in the preheated oven for about 1 hour or until the internal temperature reaches 165°F (74°C).

6. Let the chicken rest for a few minutes before carving and serving.

Adjust the portions and ingredients according to your specific dietary needs. Enjoy these tasty low-FODMAP recipes for your lunches and dinners.

Recipes for main dishes, soups, salads,

Nutritious and easy-to-prepare recipes for main dishes, soups, salads, and sides:

Main Dishes:

Baked Lemon Herb Chicken:

- Rub chicken breasts with a mixture of lemon juice, olive oil, minced garlic, and herbs.
- Place the chicken in a baking dish and bake at 375°F (190°C) for 25-30 minutes, or until cooked through.
- Serve with steamed veggies and quino

Teriyaki Salmon:

- Marinate salmon fillets in a mixture of soy sauce, honey, minced ginger, and garlic for at least 30 minutes.
- Grill or bake the salmon at 400°F (200°C) for 12-15 minutes, or until it easily flakes with a fork.
- Serve with steamed brown rice and a side of roasted asparagus.

Soups:

Lentil Soup:

- Sauté diced onion, carrots, and celery in olive oil until softened.
- Add rinsed lentils, vegetable broth, diced tomatoes, and a blend of herbs and spices.
- Simmer for about 25-30 minutes until the lentils are tender.
- Season with salt and pepper. Serve hot with a sprinkle of fresh parsley.

Chicken and Vegetable Soup:

- In a pot, cook diced chicken breast with onions, garlic, and your preferred mix of vegetables (e.g., carrots, celery, bell peppers).
- Add low-sodium chicken broth and simmer until vegetables are cooked.

- Season with thyme, rosemary, salt, and pepper. Serve with whole-grain bread.

Salads:

Greek Salad:

- Toss together chopped cucumbers, cherry tomatoes, red onion, Kalamata olives, and crumbled feta cheese.
- Drizzle with olive oil and lemon juice.
- Season with dried oregano, salt, and pepper. Serve chilled.

Quinoa and Avocado Salad:

- Cook quinoa according to package instructions and let it cool.

- Mix cooked quinoa with diced avocado, cherry tomatoes, chopped cucumber, red onion, and fresh cilantro.
- Dress with a mixture of lime juice, olive oil, salt, and pepper. Serve at room temperature.

Sides:

Roasted Sweet Potato Wedges:

- Preheat the oven to 425°F (220°C). Toss sweet potato wedges in olive oil, paprika, salt, and pepper.
- Spread them in a single layer on a baking sheet and roast for 20-25 minutes until crispy.
- Serve as a healthy alternative to French fries.

Grilled Zucchini:

- Slice zucchini lengthwise into thin strips and brush with olive oil.
- Grill over medium heat for 2-3 minutes per side, until grill marks appear.
- Season with salt, pepper, and a squeeze of lemon juice.

Main Dishes:

Veggie Stir-Fry:

- Heat some sesame oil in a pan and add your favorite stir-fry vegetables like bell peppers, broccoli, carrots, snap peas, and mushrooms.
- Sauté until the vegetables are tender-crisp.
- Add a sauce made with soy sauce, ginger, garlic, and a touch of honey.
- Serve over brown rice or noodles.

Quinoa Stuffed Bell Peppers:

- In a bowl, mix cooked quinoa with black beans, diced tomatoes, corn kernels, chopped onions, and your favorite herbs and spices.
- Cut the tops off bell peppers and remove the seeds.
- Stuff the peppers with the quinoa mixture and place them in a baking dish.
- Bake at 375°F (190°C) for 25-30 minutes, or until the peppers are tender.

Soups:

Butternut Squash Soup:

- Roast butternut squash cubes with olive oil, salt, and pepper until soft and caramelized.
- Sauté onions and garlic in a pot, then add the roasted squash, vegetable broth, and a pinch of nutmeg.
- Simmer for 15-20 minutes, then blend until smooth.

- Garnish with a drizzle of olive oil and a sprinkle of fresh herbs.

Tomato Basil Soup:

- Sauté chopped onions and garlic in a pot with olive oil until translucent.
- Add diced tomatoes, vegetable broth, and fresh basil leaves.
- Simmer for 15-20 minutes, then blend until smooth.
- Stir in a splash of heavy cream or coconut milk (optional). Season with salt and pepper.

Salads:

Caprese Salad:

- Arrange sliced tomatoes, fresh mozzarella cheese, and basil leaves on a platter.
- Drizzle with olive oil and balsamic glaze.

- Sprinkle with salt and pepper. Serve as a refreshing side salad.

Spinach and Strawberry Salad:

- Combine fresh baby spinach with sliced strawberries, crumbled feta cheese, and sliced almonds.
- Toss with a light vinaigrette made from olive oil, balsamic vinegar, dijon mustard, salt, and pepper.
- Optional: add grilled chicken or shrimp for a complete meal.

Sides:

Roasted Brussels Sprouts:

- Toss halved Brussels sprouts with olive oil, salt, and black pepper.

- Roast in the oven at 425°F (220°C) for 20-25 minutes, until crispy and golden.
- Optional: drizzle with balsamic glaze or sprinkle with grated Parmesan cheese.

Quinoa Pilaf:

- Sauté chopped onions and minced garlic in a pot with olive oil until softened.
- Add rinsed quinoa, vegetable broth, and a bay leaf.
- Simmer covered for 15-20 minutes until the quinoa is cooked and fluffy.
- Stir in toasted pine nuts or chopped almonds, along with fresh herbs like parsley or cilantro.

Feel free to adjust these recipes based on your preferences and dietary needs. Enjoy preparing these nutritious and delicious meals.

Main Dishes:

Veggie Stir-Fry:

- Heat some sesame oil in a pan and add your favorite stir-fry vegetables like bell peppers, broccoli, carrots, snap peas, and mushrooms.
- Sauté until the vegetables are tender-crisp.
- Add a sauce made with soy sauce, ginger, garlic, and a touch of honey.
- Serve over brown rice or noodles.

Quinoa Stuffed Bell Peppers:

- In a bowl, mix cooked quinoa with black beans, diced tomatoes, corn kernels, chopped onions, and your favorite herbs and spices.
- Cut the tops off bell peppers and remove the seeds.
- Stuff the peppers with the quinoa mixture and place them in a baking dish.

- Bake at 375°F (190°C) for 25-30 minutes, or
  until the peppers are tender.

Soups:

Butternut Squash Soup:

- Roast butternut squash cubes with olive oil, salt,
  and pepper until soft and caramelized.
- Sauté onions and garlic in a pot, then add the
  roasted squash, vegetable broth, and a pinch of
  nutmeg.
- Simmer for 15-20 minutes, then blend until
  smooth.
- Garnish with a drizzle of olive oil and a sprinkle
  of fresh herbs.

Tomato Basil Soup:

- Sauté chopped onions and garlic in a pot with
  olive oil until translucent.

- Add diced tomatoes, vegetable broth, and fresh basil leaves.

- Simmer for 15-20 minutes, then blend until smooth.

- Stir in a splash of heavy cream or coconut milk (optional). Season with salt and pepper.

Salads:

Caprese Salad:

- Arrange sliced tomatoes, fresh mozzarella cheese, and basil leaves on a platter.

- Drizzle with olive oil and balsamic glaze.

- Sprinkle with salt and pepper. Serve as a refreshing side salad.

Spinach and Strawberry Salad:

- Combine fresh baby spinach with sliced strawberries, crumbled feta cheese, and sliced almonds.

- Toss with a light vinaigrette made from olive oil, balsamic vinegar, dijon mustard, salt, and pepper.
- Optional: add grilled chicken or shrimp for a complete meal.

Sides:

Roasted Brussels Sprouts:

- Toss halved Brussels sprouts with olive oil, salt, and black pepper.
- Roast in the oven at 425°F (220°C) for 20-25 minutes, until crispy and golden.
- Optional: drizzle with balsamic glaze or sprinkle with grated Parmesan cheese.

Quinoa Pilaf:

- Sauté chopped onions and minced garlic in a pot with olive oil until softened.

- Add rinsed quinoa, vegetable broth, and a bay leaf.
- Simmer covered for 15-20 minutes until the quinoa is cooked and fluffy.
- Stir in toasted pine nuts or chopped almonds, along with fresh herbs like parsley or cilantro.

Feel free to adjust these recipes based on your preferences and dietary needs. Enjoy preparing these nutritious and delicious meals.

Ingredients to cater to different dietary preferences (e.g., vegetarian, gluten-free, etc.)

list of low-FODMAP ingredients that can cater to various dietary preferences, including vegetarian and gluten-free options:

Vegetables: Incorporate low-FODMAP vegetables such as bell peppers, carrots, spinach, zucchini, eggplant, tomatoes, cucumber, and lettuce. These can be used in salads, stir-fries, or roasted dishes.

Fruits: Opt for low-FODMAP fruits like strawberries, blueberries, oranges, grapes, and pineapple. These can be included in smoothies, fruit salads, or enjoyed as a snack.

Grains: Gluten-free options like rice, quinoa, buckwheat, and oatmeal can be used as a base for meals like risottos, grain bowls, or breakfast porridge.

Proteins: For vegetarian preferences, incorporate tofu, tempeh, or plant-based protein sources like lentils, chickpeas, and beans. Animal-based proteins such as chicken, turkey, fish, eggs, and seafood are also low-FODMAP options.

Nuts and seeds: Include low-FODMAP options like almonds, walnuts, chia seeds, sesame seeds, and flaxseeds. These can be sprinkled over salads, added to smoothies, or used in baking recipes.

Dairy alternatives: If catering to lactose-free preferences, utilize low-FODMAP dairy alternatives like lactose-free milk, coconut milk, almond milk, or soy milk. These can be used in cooking, baking, or enjoyed as a beverage.

Herbs and spices: Incorporate low-FODMAP herbs and spices to add flavor, such as basil, oregano, rosemary, thyme, turmeric, cumin, and paprika. These can enhance the taste of various dishes without triggering FODMAP intolerance.

Condiments: Choose low-FODMAP options like mustard, maple syrup, rice vinegar, balsamic vinegar, soy sauce (gluten-free), and olive oil for dressings, marinades, or flavoring dishes.

it's essential to check specific dietary restrictions and preferences of individuals to ensure their needs are met. By incorporating these low-FODMAP ingredients, you can create a variety of delicious, satisfying meals to cater to different dietary preferences.

SNACKS AND APPETIZERS

Low-FODMAP snack and appetizer recipes

Delicious and easy low-FODMAP snack and appetizer recipes perfect for on-the-go or entertaining guests:

Zucchini and Parmesan Fritters:

Ingredients:

- 2 medium zucchinis (grated),
- 1/4 cup grated Parmesan cheese,
- 1/4 cup gluten-free breadcrumbs,
- 2 green onions (green parts only, chopped),
- 1 egg (beaten), salt, and pepper.

Instructions:

Mix all the ingredients in a bowl. Heat a pan with oil over medium heat. Spoon the mixture onto the pan to form fritters. Cook for a few minutes on each side until golden brown. Serve warm.

Caprese Skewers:

- Ingredients: Cherry tomatoes, fresh mozzarella balls (bocconcini), fresh basil leaves, olive oil, balsamic glaze, salt, and pepper.
- Instructions: Thread cherry tomatoes, mozzarella balls, and basil leaves onto skewers. Drizzle with olive oil and balsamic glaze. Sprinkle with salt and pepper. Serve as is or marinate for a few hours for enhanced flavors.

Cucumber Sushi Rolls:

Ingredients:

- 1 large cucumber,

- 4-5 slices of cooked chicken or turkey (low-FODMAP),

- 1 red bell pepper (thinly sliced),

- 1 carrot (thinly sliced),

- 2-3 green onions (green parts only, sliced), gluten-free soy sauce (low-FODMAP version).

Instructions:

Slice the cucumber lengthwise into thin strips using a vegetable peeler. Lay one cucumber strip on a flat surface and place a slice of chicken or turkey on it. Add a few slices of bell pepper, carrot, and green onion. Roll tightly and secure with toothpicks. Repeat for the remaining ingredients. Serve with soy sauce for dipping.

Bacon-Wrapped Shrimp:

- Ingredients: Large shrimp (peeled and deveined), bacon (cut into strips), olive oil, salt, and pepper.

- Instructions: Preheat the oven to 400°F (200°C). Wrap each shrimp with a strip of bacon and secure with a toothpick. Place the wrapped shrimp on a baking sheet. Drizzle with olive oil, season with salt and pepper. Bake for 10-15 minutes until the bacon is crispy and the shrimp is cooked through. Serve hot as an appetizer.

Spinach and Feta Stuffed Mushrooms:

Ingredients:

- Medium-sized mushrooms,
- fresh spinach (chopped),
- crumbled feta cheese,
- garlic-infused olive oil,
- dried oregano, salt, and pepper.

Instructions:

Preheat the oven to 375°F (190°C). Remove the stems from the mushrooms and set aside. Place mushroom caps on a baking sheet. In a bowl, mix spinach, feta, chopped mushroom stems, garlic-infused olive oil, oregano, salt, and pepper. Spoon the mixture into the mushroom caps. Bake for 15-20 minutes until the mushrooms are tender. Serve warm.

Smoked Salmon Cucumber Bites:

Ingredients:

English cucumber, smoked salmon slices, dairy-free cream cheese (low-FODMAP), fresh dill, and lemon zest.

Instructions:

Slice the cucumber into rounds. Spread a thin layer of cream cheese on each cucumber slice. Top with a small piece of smoked salmon. Garnish with fresh dill and a sprinkle of lemon zest. Serve chilled.

Mini Chicken Lettuce Wraps:

Ingredients:

Ground chicken, lettuce leaves (such as butter lettuce or iceberg lettuce), carrots (julienned), cucumber (julienned), green onions (green parts only, sliced), gluten-free soy sauce (low-FODMAP version), sesame oil, and lime wedges.

Instructions:

In a pan, cook the ground chicken until browned. Add soy sauce, sesame oil, and green onions. Stir until well combined. Remove from heat. Take individual lettuce leaves and spoon some chicken mixture onto each leaf. Top with julienned carrots and cucumber. Squeeze lime juice on top. Roll up and secure with toothpicks. Serve as a light and refreshing appetizer.

Herbed Goat Cheese Stuffed Mini Peppers:

Ingredients:

Mini bell peppers, herbed goat cheese (ensure it's made with lactose-free ingredients), fresh herbs (such as basil, chives, or parsley, chopped), olive oil, salt, and pepper.

Instructions:

Preheat the oven to 400°F (200°C). Slice the tops off the mini peppers and remove the seeds. In a bowl, mix the herbed goat cheese, fresh herbs, salt, and pepper. Stuff each mini pepper with the cheese mixture. Place on a baking sheet and drizzle with olive oil. Bake for 10-15 minutes until the peppers are slightly softened and the cheese is melted. Serve warm or at room temperature.

Crispy Baked Kale Chips:

Ingredients:

Fresh kale leaves (stems removed and torn into pieces), olive oil, salt, and pepper.

Instructions:

Preheat the oven to 350°F (175°C). Toss the kale leaves in olive oil, salt, and pepper, ensuring they are well coated. Spread the leaves in a single layer on a baking sheet. Bake for 10-15 minutes until crispy and slightly browned. Allow them to cool before serving. These crunchy chips are a healthy and flavorful snack option.

Mediterranean Hummus Cups:

Ingredients:

Gluten-free hummus (check for low-FODMAP ingredients), cherry tomatoes (halved), cucumber (diced), Kalamata olives (pitted and chopped), fresh parsley (chopped), olive oil, lemon juice, salt, and pepper.

Instructions:

In small cups or bowls, spoon a dollop of hummus. Top with cherry tomatoes, diced cucumber, chopped olives, and fresh parsley. Drizzle with olive oil and lemon juice. Season with salt and pepper. Serve with gluten-free crackers or vegetable sticks for dipping.

These recipes will help you create a tasty selection of low-FODMAP snacks and appetizers that are perfect for on-the-go or entertaining guests. Enjoy.

Easy-to-make snacks like energy balls, vegetable sticks with dip, and gluten-free crackers

Easy-to-make snacks that are suitable for the low FODMAP diet:

- Rice cakes with almond butter: Spread a thin layer of almond butter on rice cakes for a quick and satisfying snack.

- Popcorn: Air-popped popcorn is a great low-FODMAP snack. Season it with herbs and spices like dried oregano, paprika, or nutritional yeast for added flavor.

- Greek yogurt with berries: Enjoy lactose-free Greek yogurt with a handful of fresh berries for a protein-packed snack.

- Cucumber and carrot sticks with hummus: Slice cucumbers and carrots into sticks and pair them with a low-FODMAP hummus made from chickpeas, olive oil, lemon juice, and spices.

- Banana and peanut butter: Slice a ripe banana and spread some peanut butter on each slice for a delicious and energy-boosting snack.

- Quinoa salad: Cook quinoa and mix it with chopped vegetables like bell peppers, cucumber, and zucchini. Toss with lemon juice, olive oil, and fresh herbs for a refreshing snack.

- Trail mix: Create your own low-FODMAP trail mix by combining various nuts (e.g., almonds, walnuts, or macadamia nuts), seeds (e.g., pumpkin or sunflower seeds), and dried fruits (e.g., cranberries or coconut flakes).

- Smoothies: Blend lactose-free milk with low-FODMAP fruits like berries, pineapple, or banana for a nutritious and filling snack.

- Rice paper rolls: Fill rice paper sheets with low-FODMAP vegetables such as lettuce, cucumber, and carrot. Dip them in a low-FODMAP sauce like tamari or a peanut sauce made with peanut butter, rice vinegar, and ginger.

- Baked potato chips: Thinly slice potatoes and bake them with a drizzle of olive oil until crispy. Season with salt, paprika, or other low-FODMAP spices.

- Chia seed pudding: Mix chia seeds with lactose-free milk and a low-FODMAP sweetener like maple syrup or stevia. Let it sit in the fridge overnight for a creamy and nutritious snack.

- Roasted chickpeas: Drain and rinse canned chickpeas, then toss them with olive oil, salt, and spices like cumin or paprika. Roast in the oven until crispy for a protein-rich snack.

- Sliced deli meat roll-ups: Take low-FODMAP deli meats like turkey or chicken and roll them up with lactose-free cheese, cucumber sticks, or lettuce leaves for a quick and satisfying snack.

- Nori wraps: Fill sheets of nori seaweed with low-FODMAP ingredients like sliced cucumber, avocado, and cooked shrimp or chicken. Roll them up and enjoy as a light snack.

- Edamame: Steam or boil a handful of edamame pods until tender. Sprinkle with salt for a nutritious and low-FODMAP snack packed with protein.

- Dark chocolate and almond clusters: Melt dark chocolate and mix it with whole almonds. Spoon the mixture into small clusters on parchment paper and let them cool for a rich and indulgent snack.

- Coconut yogurt with granola: Enjoy low-FODMAP coconut milk yogurt topped with a portion-controlled amount of low-FODMAP granola for a crunchy and satisfying treat.

- Stuffed bell peppers: Slice mini bell peppers in half, remove the seeds, and fill them with lactose-free cream cheese or a low-FODMAP dip like tzatziki. Enjoy as a colorful and flavorful snack.

- Oatmeal cookies: Bake gluten-free, low-FODMAP oatmeal cookies using rolled oats, mashed bananas, and a low-FODMAP sweetener like maple syrup. They make a delightful snack on-the-go.

- Veggie sushi rolls: Create sushi rolls using low-FODMAP vegetables like cucumber, bell peppers, and carrots. Use gluten-free sushi rice and nori sheets for a fun and nutritious snack.

These snack ideas should help you stay satisfied throughout the day while following a low-FODMAP diet. Remember to check food labels and ingredient lists to ensure they align with your dietary needs. Enjoy your snacks!

DESSERTS AND TREATS

Low-FODMAP desserts and treats

Following a low FODMAP diet doesn't mean you have to give up on delicious desserts and treats.

Some ideas for low FODMAP desserts that will satisfy your sweet cravings:

Chocolate Banana Smoothie:

- lend 1 ripe banana,
- 1 tablespoon of cocoa powder,
- 1 cup of lactose-free milk (or almond milk), and a handful of ice cubes.
- Enjoy this creamy and chocolaty smoothie guilt-free.

Raspberry Chia Pudding:

- Combine 1 cup of lactose-free yogurt,

- 2 tablespoons of chia seeds,

- 1/2 cup of raspberries,

- 1 tablespoon of maple syrup (if desired for extra sweetness) in a jar.

- Stir well and refrigerate overnight.

The chia seeds will absorb the liquid and create a pudding-like texture.

Coconut Macaroons:

In a bowl,

- mix 2 cups of shredded coconut,

- 1/2 cup of maple syrup,

- 2 tablespoons of coconut flour,

- 1/4 cup of melted coconut oil,

- 1 teaspoon of vanilla extract.

Using your hands, form small macaroon shapes and place them on a baking sheet lined with parchment paper. Bake at 350°F (175°C) for 12-15 minutes, or until golden brown.

Peanut Butter Energy Balls:

In a large bowl,

- combine 1 cup of gluten-free oats,
- 1/2 cup of natural peanut butter,
- 1/4 cup of maple syrup,
- 1/4 cup of chopped peanuts,
- 1/4 cup of dark chocolate chips.

Mix well, then roll the mixture into small balls. Refrigerate for 30 minutes before serving.

Grilled Pineapple with Cinnamon:

Cut a fresh pineapple into slices and sprinkle them with ground cinnamon. Grill the pineapple slices until they are tender and slightly caramelized. Serve as is, or pair with lactose-free yogurt or a scoop of dairy-free ice cream.

Blueberry Oat Crumble:

Mix 2 cups of fresh blueberries with

- 1 tablespoon of maple syrup and spread them in a baking dish. In a separate bowl, combine 1 cup of gluten-free oats,

- 1/4 cup of almond flour,

- 2 tablespoons of melted coconut oil, and a pinch of cinnamon. Crumble this mixture over the berries and bake at 375°F (190°C) for 25-30 minutes, or until the topping is golden brown.

Lemon Poppy Seed Muffins:

- In a mixing bowl, combine 1 cup of gluten-free flour, 1/4 cup of almond flour, 1/4 cup of melted coconut oil, 1/4 cup of maple syrup, 2 tablespoons of poppy seeds, 1 tablespoon of lemon zest, 1 teaspoon of baking powder, and a pinch of salt. Mix until well combined. Spoon the batter into muffin cups and bake at 350°F (175°C) for 18-20 minutes, or until a toothpick inserted comes out clean.

Dark Chocolate Bark:

- Melt dark chocolate (at least 70% cocoa) using a double boiler or microwave. Spread the melted chocolate onto a baking sheet lined with parchment paper. Sprinkle with FODMAP-friendly toppings like crushed almonds, shredded coconut, or dried cranberries (in small amounts). Allow the chocolate to set in the refrigerator, then break it into pieces for a tasty, indulgent treat.

Vanilla Berry Parfait:

- Layer lactose-free yogurt, fresh sliced strawberries, and blueberries in a glass or jar. Drizzle with a small amount of maple syrup and sprinkle with a handful of gluten-free granola or toasted oats for added crunch. Repeat the layers, ending with a dollop of yogurt on top.

-

Pumpkin Pie Smoothie:

- Blend 1/2 cup of canned pumpkin puree, 1 cup of lactose-free milk (or almond milk), 1 tablespoon of maple syrup, 1 teaspoon of pumpkin pie spice, and a handful of ice cubes.

Garnish with a sprinkle of cinnamon and nutmeg, and enjoy the fall-inspired flavors!

Almond Butter Cookies:

- In a mixing bowl, combine 1 cup of almond butter, 1/4 cup of maple syrup, 1/4 cup of almond flour, 1 teaspoon of vanilla extract, and a pinch of salt. Mix until well combined, then roll into small balls and place them on a baking sheet lined with parchment paper. Press down on each ball with a fork to create a crisscross pattern. Bake at 350°F (175°C) for 10-12 minutes or until lightly golden.

Remember to enjoy these desserts and treats in moderation and listen to your body's response. Everyone's tolerances to FODMAPs can vary, so it's essential to find your personal level of tolerance.

Recipes for indulgent desserts, such as a FODMAP-friendly chocolate cake, fruit crumble, and dairy-free ice cream options

Recipes for a FODMAP-friendly chocolate cake, fruit crumble, and dairy-free ice cream options that indulge your sweet tooth:

FODMAP-Friendly Chocolate Cake:

Ingredients:

- 1 cup gluten-free flour (such as rice flour)

- 1/2 cup unsweetened cocoa powder

- 1/2 teaspoon baking soda

- 1/2 teaspoon baking powder

- 1/4 teaspoon salt

- 1/2 cup coconut oil, melted

- 1/2 cup maple syrup

- 3/4 cup lactose-free milk (such as almond milk)

- 2 eggs

- 1 teaspoon vanilla extract

Instructions:

1. Preheat the oven to 350°F (175°C) and grease a round cake pan.

2. In a mixing bowl, whisk together the gluten-free flour, cocoa powder, baking soda, baking powder, and salt.

3. In another bowl, mix the melted coconut oil, maple syrup, lactose-free milk, eggs, and vanilla extract.

4. Gradually add the dry ingredients to the wet ingredients, whisking until well combined.

5. Pour the batter into the prepared cake pan and smooth the top.

6. Bake for 25-30 minutes or until a toothpick inserted into the center comes out clean.

7. Allow the cake to cool completely before serving or frosting.

Fruit Crumble:

Ingredients:

- 4 cups mixed berries (blueberries, raspberries, strawberries)

- 2 tablespoons maple syrup

- 1 cup gluten-free oats

- 1/2 cup almond flour

- 1/4 cup chopped pecans

- 1/4 cup coconut oil, melted

- 2 tablespoons maple syrup

- 1 teaspoon vanilla extract

- Pinch of salt

Instructions:

1. Preheat the oven to 375°F (190°C) and lightly grease a baking dish.

2. In a bowl, toss the mixed berries with 2 tablespoons of maple syrup and spread them evenly in the baking dish.

3. In a separate bowl, combine the oats, almond flour, chopped pecans, melted coconut oil, maple syrup, vanilla extract, and salt. Mix until crumbly.

4. Sprinkle the crumble mixture evenly over the berries.

5. Bake for 25-30 minutes or until the top is golden brown and the fruit is bubbling.

6. Serve warm with your favorite lactose-free ice cream.

Dairy-Free Ice Cream:

Ingredients:

- 2 cans full-fat coconut milk

- 1/2 cup maple syrup

- 1 teaspoon vanilla extract

- Optional: Flavorings like 1/2 cup cocoa powder, fruit puree, or crushed nuts

Instructions:

1. In a blender or food processor, combine the coconut milk, maple syrup, vanilla extract, and any optional flavorings. Blend until smooth.

2. Pour the mixture into an ice cream maker and churn according to the manufacturer's instructions.

3. Transfer the churned ice cream to a lidded container and freeze for at least 4 hours or until firm.

4. Serve in bowls or cones and enjoy your dairy-free ice cream.

These recipes should satisfy your craving for indulgent desserts while fitting into a FODMAP-friendly diet and dairy-free lifestyle. Enjoy!

Vegan Chocolate Mousse:

Ingredients:

- 1 ripe avocado

- 1/4 cup unsweetened cocoa powder

- 1/4 cup maple syrup

- 1/4 cup coconut milk

- 1 teaspoon vanilla extract

- Pinch of salt

Instructions:

1. Scoop the avocado flesh into a blender or food processor.

2. Add cocoa powder, maple syrup, coconut milk, vanilla extract, and salt.

3. Blend until smooth and creamy.

4. Transfer the mousse into serving dishes and refrigerate for at least 2 hours before serving.

5. Garnish with berries or coconut flakes, if desired.

Gluten-Free Apple Crisp:

Ingredients:

- 4-5 medium apples, peeled, cored, and sliced

- 1 tablespoon lemon juice

- 1/4 cup maple syrup

- 1 teaspoon ground cinnamon

- 1/2 cup gluten-free oats

- 1/4 cup almond flour

- 1/4 cup chopped walnuts

- 2 tablespoons coconut oil, melted

- 2 tablespoons maple syrup

Instructions:

1. Preheat the oven to 375°F (190°C) and lightly grease a baking dish.

2. In a bowl, toss the apple slices with lemon juice, maple syrup, and cinnamon. Transfer the mixture to the prepared baking dish.

3. In a separate bowl, combine oats, almond flour, chopped walnuts, melted coconut oil, and maple syrup. Mix until crumbly.

4. Sprinkle the crumble mixture evenly over the apples.

5. Bake for 30-35 minutes or until the top is golden brown and the apples are tender.

6. Allow it to cool for a few minutes before serving. Serve warm with dairy-free vanilla ice cream or whipped coconut cream.

Dairy-Free Chocolate Banana Nice Cream:

Ingredients:

- 3 ripe bananas, peeled and frozen

- 2 tablespoons unsweetened cocoa powder

- 2 tablespoons almond butter

- 1 teaspoon vanilla extract

- Optional toppings: chopped nuts, shredded coconut, or dairy-free chocolate chips

Instructions:

1. Place the frozen bananas, cocoa powder, almond butter, and vanilla extract in a blender or food processor.

2. Blend until smooth and creamy, scraping down the sides as needed.

3. Transfer the mixture into a lidded container and freeze for about 1 hour or until firm.

4. Serve in bowls or cones, and sprinkle with your favorite toppings.

Enjoy these delectable dessert recipes that are both delicious and suitable for your dietary preferences!

MEAL PLANS AND PREPARATION TIPS

Low-FODMAP meal plans for different dietary needs (e.g., week-long plans, vegetarian plans, etc.)

Ready-to-follow Low-FODMAP meal plans for different dietary needs:

Week-Long Low-FODMAP Meal Plan:

Day 1:

- Breakfast: Scrambled eggs with spinach and tomatoes

- Snack: Carrot sticks with lactose-free yogurt dip

- Lunch: Grilled chicken salad with mixed greens, cucumbers, and balsamic vinegar dressing

- Snack: Rice cakes with peanut butter

- Dinner: Baked salmon with roasted low-FODMAP vegetables (such as zucchini, bell peppers, and carrots)

Day 2:

- Breakfast: Quinoa porridge with almond milk, topped with strawberries and a sprinkle of almonds

- Snack: Banana with almond butter

- Lunch: Turkey lettuce wraps with low-FODMAP veggies (like bell peppers, carrots, and cucumber)

- Snack: Rice crackers with lactose-free cheese slices

- Dinner: Grilled steak with a side of steamed asparagus and mashed potatoes (made with lactose-free milk)

Day 3:

- Breakfast: Overnight oats made with gluten-free oats, lactose-free yogurt, and blueberries

- Snack: Mixed nuts

- Lunch: Grilled chicken with gluten-free pasta (made from rice or quinoa) and low-FODMAP tomato sauce

- Snack: Rice cakes with sliced avocado

- Dinner: Stir-fried tofu with bok choy and bell peppers, served over brown rice

Repeat the above menu for the remaining days of the week or mix and match according to your preferences.

Vegetarian Low-FODMAP Meal Plan:

Day 1:

- Breakfast: Vegan protein smoothie with spinach, almond milk, low-FODMAP berries, and a scoop of vegan protein powder

- Snack: Rice cakes with almond butter

- Lunch: Quinoa salad with cherry tomatoes, cucumber, black olives, and a lemon-olive oil dressing

- Snack: Low-FODMAP fruit salad (such as grapes, kiwi, and oranges)

- Dinner: Lentil curry with coconut milk, served with a side of steamed green beans and quinoa

Day 2:

- Breakfast: Vegan tofu scramble with spinach, bell peppers, and gluten-free toast

- Snack: Carrot sticks with hummus

- Lunch: Zucchini noodles with low-FODMAP pesto sauce and cherry tomatoes

- Snack: Rice crackers with sliced avocado

- Dinner: Baked tofu with roasted low-FODMAP vegetables (such as eggplant, bell peppers, and carrots)

Day 3:

- Breakfast: Quinoa porridge made with almond milk, topped with sliced banana, and a sprinkle of chia seeds

- Snack: Mixed nuts

- Lunch: Vegan chickpea salad with cucumber, cherry tomatoes, and a lemon-tahini dressing

- Snack: Rice cakes with lactose-free yogurt dip

- Dinner: Stir-fried tempeh with bok choy, bell peppers, and gluten-free tamari, served over brown rice

Pescatarian Low-FODMAP Meal Plan:

Day 1:

- Breakfast: Smoked salmon and scrambled eggs with spinach

- Snack: Sliced cucumber with lactose-free yogurt dip

- Lunch: Tuna salad with mixed greens, cherry **tomatoes, and a lemon-dijon dressing**

- Snack: Rice cakes with smoked trout

- Dinner: Grilled shrimp skewers with roasted low-FODMAP vegetables (such as zucchini, bell peppers, and carrots)

Day 2:

- Breakfast: Omelette with feta cheese, spinach, and cherry tomatoes

- Snack: Rice crackers with lactose-free cream cheese and smoked salmon

- Lunch: Grilled fish tacos in corn tortillas with low-FODMAP slaw (like cabbage, carrots, and cilantro)

- Snack: Mixed nuts

- Dinner: Baked cod with roasted asparagus and quinoa

Day 3:

- Breakfast: Greek yogurt with low-FODMAP granola and blueberries

- Snack: Seaweed snacks

- Lunch: Grilled salmon salad with mixed greens, cucumber, and lemon-olive oil dressing

- Snack: Rice cakes with tuna salad

- Dinner: Sautéed scallops with zucchini noodles and a low-FODMAP tomato sauce

Vegan Low-FODMAP Meal Plan:

Day 1:

- Breakfast: Vegan protein smoothie bowl with almond milk, low-FODMAP berries, and a sprinkle of chia seeds

- Snack: Rice cakes with almond butter

- Lunch: Quinoa and roasted vegetable salad with cherry tomatoes and a lemon-tahini dressing

- Snack: Low-FODMAP fruit salad (such as grapes, kiwi, and oranges)

- Dinner: Vegan lentil and vegetable curry with coconut milk, served with brown rice

Day 2:

- Breakfast: Chia seed pudding with almond milk, topped with sliced banana and crushed walnuts

- Snack: Carrot sticks with hummus

- Lunch: Tofu stir-fry with bell peppers, bok choy, and gluten-free tamari, served over rice noodles

- Snack: Rice crackers with sliced avocado

- Dinner: Vegan chickpea and vegetable stew with a side of quinoa

Day 3:

- Breakfast: Gluten-free oatmeal topped with low-FODMAP berries, coconut flakes, and a drizzle of maple syrup

- Snack: Mixed nuts

- Lunch: Zucchini and carrot noodles with low-FODMAP pesto sauce and cherry tomatoes

- Snack: Rice cakes with lactose-free yogurt dip

- Dinner: Vegan tempeh stir-fry with broccoli, bell peppers, and gluten-free tamari, served over brown rice

Remember, these meal plans are just a starting point, and you can customize them according to your preferences and dietary needs

Strategies for meal prepping and batch cooking

Strategies to help you with meal prepping and batch cooking for a Low-FODMAP diet:

Plan your meals: Take some time each week to plan your meals in advance. Look for Low-FODMAP recipes and design a meal plan that includes a variety of foods while keeping your dietary restrictions in mind.

Make a shopping list: Once you have your meal plan, create a shopping list that includes all the ingredients you'll need. This will prevent you from buying unnecessary items and ensure you have everything you need for your meal prep.

Prep your ingredients: Before you start cooking, do some prep work. Chop vegetables, wash and cut fruits, and measure out spices and other ingredients. Having everything ready beforehand will help streamline the cooking process.

Cook in batches: Batch cooking is a great way to save time and ensure you have ready-to-eat meals throughout the week. Prepare larger quantities of your chosen recipes and divide them into individual portions. You can store them in airtight containers in the fridge or freezer for easy access later.

Use versatile ingredients: Choose ingredients that can be used in multiple dishes to save time and reduce waste. For example, roast a big batch of chicken or prepare a large pot of rice that can be used as a base for different meals.

Utilize slow cookers or instant pots: These appliances can be a game-changer for meal prepping. You can set them up in the morning with your chosen ingredients, and by the end of the day, you'll have a delicious meal ready to be portioned out for the week.

Pre-portion your meals: Divide your cooked meals into individual portions in appropriate-sized containers. This will make it easy to grab a meal when you're in a hurry, and you won't be tempted to eat more than you planned.

Freeze meals for later: If you're not planning to eat the meals within a few days, freezing them is a great option. Just make sure to label the containers with the meal name and date before freezing for easier organization.

Experiment with spices and herbs: Low-FODMAP doesn't mean your food has to be bland. Experiment with different herbs, spices, and seasonings to add flavor to your meals without triggering any digestive issues.

Keep snacks on hand: Prepare Low-FODMAP snacks in advance, such as veggie sticks, rice cakes, or homemade trail mix. This will ensure you have suitable options available when you need a quick bite.

Remember, always consult with a healthcare professional or dietitian to ensure you're following a Low-FODMAP diet correctly and that it meets your specific dietary needs.

DINING OUT AND TRAVELING GUIDES

Strategies for dining out while adhering to a Low-FODMAP diet

Dining out while following a Low-FODMAP diet can be a bit challenging but with some preparation and careful choices, you can still enjoy eating out without experiencing digestive discomfort. Here are some practical advice and strategies for dining out while adhering to a Low-FODMAP diet:

Plan ahead: Do some research before choosing a restaurant. Look for menus online or call ahead to inquire about low-FODMAP options. This will help you select the best possible restaurant for your dietary needs.

Communicate your dietary requirements: Inform the waiter or server about your diet restrictions. Clearly explain that you are following a Low-FODMAP diet and ask for their assistance in selecting suitable dishes or making modifications if necessary. Most restaurants are accommodating and will be happy to accommodate your needs.

Be cautious with sauces and dressings: Many sauces and dressings used in restaurants can contain high-FODMAP ingredients like garlic, onion, or honey. Ask for dressings and sauces on the side so you can control the amount you consume, or request them to be made without high-FODMAP ingredients.

Choose simple, whole food options: Opt for dishes that contain simple, low-FODMAP ingredients such as grilled meat or fish, plain rice, steamed vegetables, or salads without high-FODMAP components like onions or garlic. These options are usually safer and easier to customize if needed.

Avoid hidden FODMAPs: Stay away from dishes that commonly contain FODMAP-rich ingredients like wheat, high-lactose dairy, legumes, garlic, or onion. Be cautious with soups, stews, gravies, and marinades, as they often contain hidden FODMAPs.

Ask about cooking methods: Inquire about how the food is prepared. Grilled, baked, or steamed dishes are generally safer options than fried or heavily seasoned ones, as they are less likely to contain high-FODMAP ingredients.

Carry a FODMAP-friendly snack: If you're unsure about the available options or you're concerned there might not be suitable choices, take a small low-FODMAP snack with you. This way, you can enjoy a snack if necessary, ensuring you don't go hungry or make poor food choices.

Be cautious with international cuisines: Different cuisines may have a higher likelihood of containing certain high-FODMAP ingredients. For example, Chinese and Thai cuisines often use garlic and onion, while Indian cuisine uses a variety of FODMAP-rich spices. Research the specific cuisine or ingredients used before visiting a restaurant.

Consider dietary supplements: If you're concerned about accidentally consuming FODMAPs while eating out, you may want to consider taking a digestive enzyme or probiotic supplement. These can help improve your digestion and reduce symptoms if you do consume small amounts of FODMAPs.

Remember, every individual's tolerance to FODMAPs varies, so it's important to pay attention to your personal triggers and adjust your selections accordingly. It's also recommended to work with a registered dietitian who specializes in the Low-FODMAP diet to get personalized guidance and support.

Navigating menus, communicating with restaurant staff

Navigating Menus:

Take your time: Carefully read through the menu to familiarize yourself with the dishes and options available. If you're unsure about something, don't hesitate to ask the staff for clarification.

Consider dietary restrictions: If you have specific dietary restrictions or allergies, look for menu items marked with symbols or keywords that indicate suitability. Many restaurants offer alternative choices for vegetarians, vegans, gluten-free, or other dietary needs.

Pay attention to dish descriptions: Menus often provide descriptions of each dish, including ingredients and preparation methods. This can help you make informed choices based on your preferences.

Ask for recommendations: Restaurant staff are usually knowledgeable about the menu and can suggest popular or specialty dishes. Don't be afraid to seek their advice if you're having trouble deciding.

Communicating with Restaurant Staff:

Be polite and respectful: Address the staff with a friendly demeanor and use "please" and "thank you" when making requests or asking questions.

Ask for clarification: If you have questions about a dish's ingredients, preparation, or portion size, feel free to ask. Staff members are there to help and can answer your queries.

Inform about allergies or dietary restrictions: If you have any food allergies or dietary restrictions, communicate this clearly to the staff. They can guide you toward suitable options or suggest modifications to meet your needs.

Seek recommendations or customization: If you need assistance in making choices, ask the staff for recommendations based on your preferences or dietary requirements. They may also be able to accommodate certain customizations to dishes.

Making Informed Food Choices:

Balance your meal: Look for options that include a variety of food groups such as protein, vegetables, whole grains, and healthy fats. This ensures a balanced and nutritious meal.

Consider portion sizes: Some restaurants offer various portion sizes or serving options. Choose a size that suits your appetite and dietary goals. If you're unsure, don't hesitate to ask the staff for guidance.

Opt for healthier preparations: Look for cooking methods like grilling, steaming, or baking, which are typically healthier choices compared to deep-frying or heavy sauces.

Mindful eating: Listen to your body's hunger and fullness cues to avoid overeating. Take your time to savor each bite and enjoy the flavors.

Remember, restaurant staff are there to assist you, so don't hesitate to ask questions or seek guidance. They want you to have an enjoyable dining experience and make informed food choices.

Traveling while on a Low-FODMAP plan and suggestions for Low-FODMAP-friendly snacks to pack

Traveling while on a low-FODMAP (Fermentable Oligosaccharides, Disaccharides, Monosaccharides, and Polyols) plan may require a bit of preparation to ensure you have access to suitable food options. Some tips for traveling on a low-FODMAP plan and some low-FODMAP-friendly snack suggestions to pack:

Research your destination: Before you travel, research restaurants and grocery stores at your destination that offer low-FODMAP food options. Look for places that offer gluten-free or allergen-free menus, as they are more likely to have suitable choices.

Pack your own snacks: It's always a good idea to pack your own low-FODMAP snacks to have on hand, especially during flights or long car journeys. This way, you won't have to rely solely on the food options available during your travel.

Prepare a meal plan: Create a meal plan for your trip, particularly for any long travel days. This will help you stay organized and ensure you have access to low-FODMAP meals along the way.

Carry a "FODMAP Friendly" card: If you're traveling to a country where English is not widely spoken, consider carrying a FODMAP-friendly card that explains your dietary restrictions in the local language. This will be helpful when communicating your needs to restaurants or food vendors.

Choose low-FODMAP snack options: Here are some low-FODMAP-friendly snacks you can pack for your trip:

- Fresh fruits: Choose low-FODMAP options such as strawberries, grapes, oranges, and kiwi (in small quantities).

- Vegetable sticks: Pack carrot sticks, cucumber slices, and bell pepper strips.

- Hard-boiled eggs: Cook some hard-boiled eggs before your trip for a protein-packed snack.

- Nuts: Opt for low-FODMAP nuts like almonds, peanuts (avoid honey-roasted variants), and macadamia nuts.

- Rice cakes: Plain rice cakes make a convenient and lightweight snack option.

- Low-FODMAP granola bars: Look for granola bars made with oats, nuts, and dried fruits that are low in FODMAPs.

- Lactose-free cheese: If you tolerate lactose, consider packing lactose-free cheese cubes or slices.

Remember to always check the ingredient labels and portion sizes when choosing snacks to ensure they are low in FODMAPs. Also, keep in mind that individual tolerance levels may vary. Consult with a registered dietitian specializing in the low-FODMAP diet for personalized advice before traveling.

CONCLUSION AND MAINTENANCE TIPS

The Low-FODMAP diet is a dietary approach that has gained popularity in managing digestive conditions such as irritable bowel syndrome (IBS). It is based on limiting dietary fermentable carbohydrates (FODMAPs), which can trigger symptoms like bloating, gas, and abdominal pain in susceptible individuals. Here are the key takeaways from the book emphasizing the importance of long-term adherence to the Low-FODMAP diet for optimal digestive health:

Identification of trigger foods: The Low-FODMAP diet aims to identify specific foods that may exacerbate digestive symptoms. By following the diet strictly for a few weeks and then gradually reintroducing different FODMAP groups, individuals can pinpoint the specific triggers that affect their digestive health.

Symptom reduction: The primary goal of the Low-FODMAP diet is to reduce symptoms related to IBS, such as bloating, diarrhea, and constipation. Research has shown that a significant number of individuals experience symptom improvement on this diet. However, adherence is crucial for long-term relief.

Individualized approach: The Low-FODMAP diet recognizes that trigger foods can vary from person to person. What may cause symptoms for one individual may be well-tolerated by another. By identifying individual triggers and tailoring the diet accordingly, long-term symptom management can be achieved.

Nutritional balance: While the Low-FODMAP diet restricts certain fermentable carbohydrates, it's important to ensure nutritional adequacy. The book emphasizes the importance of consulting a healthcare professional or registered dietitian to ensure proper nutrient intake by incorporating suitable alternatives and understanding portion sizes.

Reintroduction phase: After the initial elimination phase, the book emphasizes the significance of the reintroduction phase. This involves systematically reintroducing specific FODMAP groups to determine personal tolerance levels. It helps expand the variety of foods in the long term while reducing unnecessary dietary restrictions.

Long-term adherence: The book underscores the importance of maintaining a long-term commitment to the Low-FODMAP diet for optimal digestive health. While strict adherence may be necessary initially, individuals are encouraged to personalize their diet to minimize restrictions while avoiding trigger foods.

By following these key takeaways and committing to long-term adherence to the Low-FODMAP diet, individuals with IBS or digestive conditions can experience significant symptom relief, improve their quality of life, and better understand their individual needs and triggers for optimal digestive health.

APPENDIX:

Low-FODMAP ingredients and their alternatives

Vegetables:

- Low-FODMAP options: spinach, kale, bok choy, cucumber, carrot, bell peppers, zucchini, eggplant, tomatoes, green beans.

- Alternatives: Avoid high-FODMAP vegetables such as onion, garlic, mushrooms, cauliflower, asparagus, and peas. Instead, consider using garlic-infused oil for flavor or use the green part of spring onions.

Fruits:

- Low-FODMAP options: strawberries, blueberries, grapes, oranges, kiwi, pineapple, honeydew melon.

- Alternatives: Limit high-FODMAP fruits like apples, pears, peaches, cherries, watermelon, and mangoes. Opt for small servings of bananas or opt for low-FODMAP fruit juices.

Grains:

- Low-FODMAP options: rice (white, brown), quinoa, oats, gluten-free bread, gluten-free pasta (made from rice or corn).

- Alternatives: Avoid wheat- and rye-based products, as they contain high-FODMAPs. Look for gluten-free options or those made with alternative grains like corn or buckwheat.

Proteins:

- Low-FODMAP options: chicken, turkey, beef, pork, tofu, tempeh, seafood (fish, shrimp, scallops), eggs.

- Alternatives: Many proteins are naturally low-FODMAP, but be cautious of added seasonings or sauces that may contain high-FODMAP ingredients like garlic or onion.

Dairy:

- Low-FODMAP options: lactose-free milk, lactose-free yogurt, lactose-free cheese (hard aged varieties like cheddar).

- Alternatives: Replace regular dairy products with lactose-free options to avoid lactose-induced symptoms. Alternatively, try non-dairy alternatives like almond milk, coconut milk, or lactose-free products made from soy.

Sweeteners:

- Low-FODMAP options: stevia, glucose, maple syrup (in moderate amounts), rice malt syrup.

- Alternatives: Avoid high-FODMAP sweeteners such as honey, agave syrup, fructose, and high fructose corn syrup. Opt for low-FODMAP sweeteners or use glucose as a substitute.

Remember, the list above is a general guideline, and individual tolerances may vary

Pantry checklist for stocking a Low-FODMAP kitchen

Stocking your pantry with low-FODMAP ingredients is a great way to ensure you have a variety of options for cooking and preparing meals while following a low-FODMAP diet. Here's a checklist to help you get started:

Grains and Bread Products:

- Gluten-free grains (rice, quinoa, oats)

- Gluten-free bread (check for no onion or garlic additives)

- Gluten-free pasta (made from rice, corn, or quinoa)

Canned and Dried Goods:

- Canned fish (tuna, salmon)

- Canned tomatoes (check for no onion or garlic additives)

- Low-FODMAP broths (vegetable, chicken, beef)

- Canned beans (lentils, chickpeas, black beans)

- Dried herbs and spices (cumin, paprika, oregano)

- Low-FODMAP sauces (soy sauce, tamari, fish sauce)

Oils and Condiments:

- Extra virgin olive oil

- Coconut oil

- Mayonnaise (check for no onion or garlic additives)

- Mustard (check for no onion or garlic additives)

- Vinegars (such as white wine vinegar, apple cider vinegar)

- Low-FODMAP salad dressings

Snacks and Spreads:

- Rice cakes

- Low-FODMAP granola bars

- Peanut or almond butter

- Rice crackers

- Popcorn (plain, unflavored)

Baking Supplies:

- Gluten-free flour (rice flour, almond flour, oat flour)

- Baking soda

- Baking powder (check for no wheat additives)

- Maple syrup or other low-FODMAP sweeteners

Nuts and Seeds:

- Almonds

- Walnuts

- Sunflower seeds

- Chia seeds

- Pumpkin seeds

Miscellaneous:

- Gluten-free soy sauce or tamari

- Low-FODMAP protein powder (if desired)

- Lactose-free or plant-based milk (such as almond or coconut milk)

- Olives and pickles (check for no onion or garlic additives)

Remember to always check labels for any hidden sources of potential high-FODMAP ingredients. It's also a good idea to consult a registered dietitian or healthcare professional for personalized advice and guidance when following a low-FODMAP diet.

www.ingramcontent.com/pod-product-compliance
Lightning Source LLC
Chambersburg PA
CBHW070837250726
48662CB00003B/1272